Dr. High Yield's
OB/GYN Notes
(for the Step 2 CK & Shelf Exams)

Steven K. M. Vuu, M.D.

DEDICATION

to all sentient beings

CONTENTS

ACKNOWLEDGMENTS

To my family (Mom, Dad, Andrew), teachers, colleagues, and all those who have helped me along the way, I wouldn't be where I am today without you. Thank you.

DR. HIGH YIELD OB/GYN NOTES

Introduction:

These are my never before seen notes I used to prepare for my Step 2 CK and shelf board examinations. It is basically a conglomeration of all the books I read and the practice questions I did during 3rd year medical school. The notes are written in a short form, casual manner, deliberately. I used it as a way to cement knowledge and maximize repetitions before the exam. Before you read this, remember that this is not meant to be a primary study resource. These notes are meant to supplement your baseline studies, you should already have an understanding of the basics. This is for a quick review of potent things you might have overlooked or forgotten. These bullet points are meant to be quickly read through. They will help you zone in on key details and equip you with knowledge to help answer a question you may encounter. It is in numbered form on purpose. This helps you keep focus and know how far along you are without losing your place in the list. It is best used as a last minute read the last few days prior to the exam where you don't have enough time to read a textbook or do more practice questions. If you are having trouble understanding, then go back to the source textbook or question bank and fill in the details as you wish. Best of luck on your exam. Enjoy!

Abbreviations:

2/2 = secondary to

a/w = associated with

r/o = rule out

CI = contraindication

tx = treatment

rx = treatment

dx = diagnosis

fx = fracture

w/u = work up

f/u = follow up

w/ = with

se = side effect

ae = adverse effect

LN = lymph node

LNopathy = lymphadenopathy

u/s or us = ultrasound

abx = antibiotics

****

Things to Keep in Mind When Doing Questions:

1. **rule out** the other answers
2. if u know one of them to be true and are unsure then **pick the one u know to be true**
3. if u dont know **pick the more common things**
4. **keep it simple**
5. if u dont know **move on quick** and take the L on that question and move on to save time and get other ones right
6. **age** is important
7. put the **whole picture** together
8. when it comes down to 2 answers, try to reject one of them

OBSTETRICS

1. postmenopausal woman with a thickened endometrial stripe is malignancy until proven otherwise
   1. if 45 yo+ = ENB
   2. if <45 + obesity = ENB
2. most common cause of postpartum hemorrhage = uterine atony
3. most common cause of postpartum hemorrhage with firm uterus = laceration
4. tubo ovarian abscess = be careful for rupture and hypotensive shock
   1. rx = metronidazole + clindamycin
   2. dx = US
5. active phase = >6cm dilation
6. early deceleration = head compression
7. delayed deceleration = hypoxia
8. recurrent delayed decelerations = fetal acidosis
9. variable deceleration = cord compression, tx = reposition
10. accelerations = increase FHR by 15 for 15 seconds
    1. normal NST = 2 accelerations in 20 mins
11. arrest of active phase = if no dilation after 4 hours with good contractions or 6 hours if given oxytocin supplementation
12. normal second stage = <3 hours (epidural is 4)
    1. if longer than 3 hours = arrest of descent = c section
13. indications for C-section = cephalopelvic disproportion, arrest of active phase, uterus rupture, prolapsed cord
14. fetal tachycardia = maternal fever
15. adequate contractions = IUPC >200 montevideo units in 10 mins or contractions every 2-3 mins lasting 40 seconds each contraction
16. montevideo units = the sum of the uterus pressure changes

above baseline with each contraction in 10 mins

17. tachysystole = 5+ uterine contractions every 10 mins rx = terbutaline/tocolytic

18. bloody show = loss of cervical mucus/blood plug red/yellow plug that is a sign of labor onset

19. ephedrine = good for maternal hypotension because it does not constrict uterine arteries

20. oxytocin does not affect cervical dilation

21. elevated Hb A2 = beta thalassemia

22. beta thalassemia major baby = healthy at birth until HbF falls

23. G6PD provoking drugs = sulfa, nitrofurantoin, antimalarials

24. dark colored urine in G6PD deficiency = bilirubinuria

25. anemia of pregnancy is due to increased plasma volume dilution of RBC concentration

26. uterine inversion leads to massive hemorrhage because it limits the uterus ability to clamp the spiral arteries

27. uterotonic agents = oxytocin, misoprostol, ergotamine/methergine
    1. methergine is 2nd line if oxytocin doesn't work

28. after 30 mins if placenta doesn't deliver, tx = manual extraction (if wait too long = hemorrhage)

29. mcroberts maneuver = flexion of hips to treat shoulder dystocia

30. prenatal risk factors for shoulder dystocia in order: prior dystocia, macrosomia, gestational diabetes

31. complications of dystocia = erb palsy, clavicle fx, hypoxia, death

32. bradycardia = less than 110 bpm for 10 mins

33. uterine rupture = u will see a very long delayed declaration

34. prolonged bradycardia = rupture, cord prolapse, tachysystole

35. maneuvers that improve delivery of o2 to the fetus:
    1. left lateral decubitus takes weight off the IVC
    2. 100% o2 for the mom

     3. give mom IV fluids

36. fetal HR acceleration = good sign of o2 for baby = if u see 15 bpm rise for 15 seconds

37. uterine rupture tx = c section

38. cord prolapse tx = c section

39. uterine atony tx = massage + oxytocin + bladder emptying

40. postpartum hemorrhage = pph = 500 ml loss +, if c section = 1 L+

41. methergine = ergot alkaloid = induces myometrial contraction
     1. CI = HTN because leads to stroke

42. prostaglandin F2 alpha =carboprost = myometrial contraction = mechanism for primary dysmenorrhea
     1. CI = Asthma
     2. this is why NSAIDS work for tx of primary dysmenorrhea

43. primary PPH = within first 24 hours

44. secondary PPH = after first 24 hours
     1. tx = methergine

45. causes of uterine atony = magnesium, rapid/long labor, overstretched uterus, multiparous, oxytocin use during labor, tired uterus

46. secondary/late PPH = subinvolution of placental site, like a scab that falls off and makes u bleed
     1. tx = ergot alkaloid aka methergine

47. retained products of conception tx = D&C

48. endometritis tx = clindamycin + gentamicin
     1. signs = uterine fundus tender, fever, foul smelling lochia
     2. lochia = postpartum discharge of blood mucus and tissue

49. non smelly lochia = normal = shedding of endometrium after pregnancy, can take weeks to finish

50. umbilicus fundal height = at week 20
51. nuchal translucency transvaginal USS = down syndrome or trisomy 18 (seen weeks 10-13)
52. >2 to 2.5 MOM (multiples of the median) = neural tube defect (NTD)
53. elevated AFP = NTD, abdominal wall defect, oligohydramnios, underestimate age
54. low AFP = overestimate age, trisomy, molar preg, fetal death
55. DS = thickened nuchal fold, nuchal translucency, short femur length, echogenic bowel for duodenal atresia
56. fetal karyotype taken thru amniocentesis
57. mtx -> limb and skeleton defects
58. retinoic acid -> face defect, NTD
59. ace inhibitor -> renal tubule dysgenesis
60. warfarin -> nerve and skeleton defect
61. most common abnormal triple screen = wrong dating
62. organogenesis = weeks 3-8
63. risk factors for vasa previa = velamentous cord insertion, accessory lobes, second trimester placenta previa, IVF
64. twins have higher rate of preterm delivery, congenital malformations, preeclampsia, PPH
65. twin twin transfusion syndrome TTT = when one twin gives all the resources to the other twin
    1. big twin = macrosomia, polycythemia, polyhydramnios, CNS problems
    2. small twin = microsomia, anemia, oligohydramnios
66. clomiphene = induces ovulation and promotes maturation of multiple follicles leading to multiple eggs being released; tx for PCOS pregnancy
67. rx for TTT = laser ablation of anastomosis vessels
68. if vasa previa identified, should have planned C-section before ROM at around 35-36 week to prevent fetus from dying

69. Kleihauer Betke test = determines dosage for rhogam
70. preeclampsia -> pulmonary edema via increased plasma volume tx = furosemide IV
71. presence of prodromal sx or genital lesions suspicious for HSV = c section
72. chancroid = ragged edges, necrotic base, adenopathy
    1. school of fish, rx = ceftriaxone and azithro
73. c section -> incr risk of placenta previa -> increased risk for placenta accreta
74. abruption complications = hemorrhage, fetal to maternal bleeding, coagulopathy, preterm delivery
75. proteinuria = P/C protein to creatinine ratio 0.3+
76. abruption risk factors = trauma, previous abruption, HTN, cocaine, submucosal leiomyoma (can peel off easier), polyhydramnios (heavy bag detaches), cigs, PPROM
77. placenta accreta rx = hysterectomy
78. accreta formed by defect in decidua basalis layer aka missing, placental villi attach to myometrium
79. placenta percreta usually invades bladder or bowel too
80. trophotropism = when the uterus expands and the placenta previa is no longer covering the cervix
81. placenta accreta is a risk factor for uterine inversion
82. placenta percreta -> bladder perforation -> hematuria
83. pregnancy -> increased biliary sludge -> gallstones -> RUQ pain following a meal
84. hcg helps keep corpus luteum alive to produce progesterone till around 10 weeks, when the placenta takes over and produces progesterone
85. intrahepatic cholestasis of pregnancy tx = ursodiol = lowers serum bile acid levels
    1. itchy at night on palms and soles
    2. LFT damage

3. increased systemic bile acid levels
4. bile salts incompletely cleared by liver -> deposit in dermis -> itchy = ICP / usually 3rd semester problem

86. PUPPP = pruritic urticarial papules and plaques of pregnancy
    1. begins in abdominal area over striae and spreads to the buttocks
    2. benign
    3. perivascular lymphocytes associated with edema of papillary dermis
    4. tx = steroids

87. herpes gestationis = bullous pemphigoid of pregnancy = vesicles on abdomen and extremities
    1. antibody vs hemidesmosomes IgG
    2. tx = corticosteroids
    3. IgG can cross placenta and baby can have transiently after birth

88. acute fatty liver of pregnancy = microvesicular steatosis of the liver = hypoglycemia + LFTs
    1. mitochondrial dysfxn in oxidation of fatty acids
    2. acute renal failure, hypoglycemia, liver failure
    3. deliver baby immediately high risk of death

89. pregnant women predisposed to DVT via IVC uterus clamping leading to stasis + lots of clotting factors -> clot formed

90. estrogen -> increased liver synthesis HIGH fibrinogen -> hypercoagulable = HIGH FIBRINOGEN

91. DVT dx = venous duplex doppler USS

92. amniotic fluid embolism = occurs during labor
    1. chest rash + fetal debris gets into maternal bloodstream
    2. a/w c section, induction of labor, abruption
    3. tx = supportive
    4. most common cause for maternal mortality = embolus into lungs

93. homozygous factor V leiden mutation = protein c resistance; tx = LMW heparin

94. PaO2 in a pregnant mom should be at least 80+ to be normal

95. chronic HTN = before pregnancy or before 20 weeks

96. gestational htn = HTN onset after 20 weeks pregnancy

97. severe feature of preeclampsia = maternal end organs threatened = MUST deliver baby

98. proteinuria definition = 300 mg of protein in 24 hours or protein to creatinine ratio of >0.3 or dipstick 1+

99. preeclampsia pulmonary edema tx = IV furosemide

100. preeclampsia bp = 140/90

101. preeclampsia with severe features = 160/110 bp + end organ damage; tx = magnesium + deliver

102. preeclampsia -> leaky vessels -> edema

103. severe preeclampsia tx = mag sulfate + deliver

104. hyporeflexia DTR first sign of toxic magnesium dose

105. pregnancy elevated LFT = preeclampsia, HELLP, ICP, acute fatty liver pregnancy

106. causes for preterm labor = UTI, STD, abruption, polyhydramnios

107. magnesium sulfate helps prevent cerebral palsy in preterm infants

108. betamethasone administration prevents RDS

109. very premature babies <28 weeks are at risk for intraventricular hemorrhage, corticosteroids help this

110. cervical length of <25 mm is at risk for preterm labor = best predictor

111. most important risk factor for preterm is prior preterm

112. tocolysis is used if baby <34 weeks

113. magnesium used up to week 32

114. betamethasone used up to week 37

115. magnesium = competitive inhibition of calcium to decrease

actin myosin interaction

116. weekly 17 hydroxyprogesterone injections = helps prevent preterm birth with women at high risk

117. TOCOLYSIS CAUSES PULMONARY EDEMA

118. tx for chorioamnionitis = IV ampicillin and gentamicin + vaginal labor

119. signs of chorioamnionitis = fever, tender uterus, fetal tachycardia

120. neonatal infections = BEL = group B strep, e coli, listeria

121. rupture of membrane (ROM) signs = gush of fluid, ferning pattern of fluid on microscopy, oligohydramnios, nitrazine test alkali pH vaginal fluid, amnisure test

122. amnisure test = alpha macroglobulin marker specific for placenta

123. marker for mature fetal lungs = PG = phosphatidylglycerol

124. confirmation of chorioamnionitis = amniotic fluid gram stain

125. chorioamnionitis without rupture = Listeria via transplacental spread, unpasteurized milk

126. PPROM -> oligohydramnios -> cord compression -> recurrent variable decelerations -> tx = mom changes position alleviates cord compression OR amnioinfusion

127. parvovirus -> inhibits fetus erythrocyte production -> aplastic crisis -> tachycardia -> heart failure -> hydrops fetalis edema -> polyhydramnios compensation (everything is swollen)

128. fetal severe anemia causes liver to pick up the slack to make RBC but then it makes less albumin and leads to anasarca

129. adult parvovirus = myalgias, arthralgias, malaise (similar to RA but transient)

130. sinusoidal heart rate pattern = sign of severe anemia or asphyxia, 3-5 sine waves per minute

131. CMV = chorioretinitis, microcephaly, ventricular

calcifications, transmission highest in 3rd semester

1. no cure
2. prevent by hand washing and not sharing utensils with kids
3. hepatosplenomegaly
4. most common perinatal infection worldwide

132. toxoplasma from undercooked meat or oocysts from cat feces

1. triad of cranial calcifications, hydrocephalus, chorioretinitis, ascites
2. mom treated with spiramycin
3. fetus treated with pyrimethamine and sulfadiazine

133. TORCHES infections are dx with serology or PCR

134. rubella triad = cataract, deafness, cardiac

1. abnormal light reflex = cataracts
2. very high vertical transmission rate in first trimester 50% chance

135. normal amniotic fluid volume = 5 to 25 cm

136. MC<u>A</u> artery doppler studies = increased flow is a sign of <u>A</u>nemia

1. <u>IU</u>GR measured with <u>U</u>mbilical artery doppler; reverse flow is a bad sign = fetal hypoxia = deliver

137. chlamydia can lead to neonatal pneumonia and conjunctivitis

138. erythromycin eye drops = only effective for gonococcus

139. erythromycin oral systemic = treatment for chlamydia conjunctivitis

140. chlamydia -> urethritis, mucopurulent cervicitis, late postpartum endometritis

141. chlamydia is most common cause of neonatal conjunctivitis

142. gonococcus = pustular skin lesions, arthralgias, septic arthritis

143. HIV mom should avoid breastfeeding cuz it can transfer thru milk
144. HIV prodromal is like mono triad = fever, sore throat, lymphadenopathy (+rash tho)
145. goal for pregnant HIV tx = <1000 RNA copies/mL
146. if viral load is 1000+ copies of RNA/ML then u should do a C-section
147. C-section for HIV mom must happen before going into labor or rupture of membrane or its too late
148. HIV vaginal delivery give zidovudine during labor and then give neonate oral zidovudine after too
149. Infant to Hep B mom should receive hep B Ig and vaccination at birth
150. HIV is often associated with Hep C in the mom up to half of all cases
151. Hep B and C breast feed is ok
152. tx for thyroid storm = beta blocker, steroids, PTU or methimazole
153. methimazole = teratogenic = cutis aplasia, avoid in 1st trimester
154. thyroid storm can reach baby and cause baby to have HF and hydrops
155. postpartum thyroiditis = similar to hashimoto but first u get hyperthyroid destruction of gland and then hypothyroid
    1. aka lymphocytic thyroiditis
    2. antithyroperoxidase and antimicrosomal
    3. risk factors = DM1 and previous postpartum thyroiditis
156. hypothyroidism in pregnancy = levothyroxine replacement in first trimester
157. normal pregnancy = increase TBG, increase total t4, same free t4; needs more thyroid replacement
158. maternal graves can cause fetal hyperthyroidism cuz the

IgG can cross the placenta

159. symmetric growth = head and body same size
    1. caused by chromosomal and TORCH congenital infection
160. asymmetric growth = head is bigger than body
    1. caused by placental insufficiency hypoxia, HTN, smoking, drugs, nutrition
161. mom factors that cause IUGR = heart, lung, kidney diseases, HTN, preeclampsia, anemia, drugs
162. uterine placental factors that cause IUGR = abruptio placentae, placenta previa, infection
163. baby factors that cause IUGR = congenital defect, infection
164. IUGR = birth weight less than 10th percentile
165. doppler flow study = umbilical artery US helpful for IUGR dx
166. reverse end diastolic flow on doppler study is associated with stillbirth within 48 hours and fetal hypoxia -> must deliver
167. dating error = if u do a follow up ultrasound and the baby is growing at a good pace, in IUGR the baby does not grow at a good pace
168. complications of IUGR = meconium aspiration, nec enterocolitis, hypoglycemia, RDS, hypothermia, thrombocytopenia
169. first step in evaluating size less than dates is to perform US for fetal height
170. umbilical artery doppler = distinguishes IUGR from small and healthy baby
171. IUGR dx = umbilical artery doppler
172. number 1 cause of UTI/pyelonephritis = e coli
173. asymptomatic bacteriuria in pregnancy is high risk for pyelonephritis, do urine culture in first trimester, give prophylactic abx

174. most common cause of post c-section fever = Endomyometritis
175. cause of endomyometritis = ascending infection of polymicrobial vaginal organisms
176. tx for endometritis = IV gentamicin + clindamycin
177. tx for pelvic thrombophlebitis = abx + IV heparin
178. breast abscess cause = s aureus
    1. tx = dicloxacillin + drainage
    2. dx = US if hard to dx
179. galactocele = collection of milk behind blocked mammary duct
    1. resolves spontaneously but may need drainage if stubborn
180. breastfeeding has all vitamins except K and D
181. mom health benefits of breastfeeding = lower cancer, lower weight, no diabetes, no osteoporosis
182. baby benefits of breastfeeding = less infections, less allergies, less diabetes, smarter, no necrotizing enterocolitis
183. HIV CI for breastfeeding
184. vitamin D should be supplemented at 2 months of age, infants should breastfeed exclusively for the first 6 months of life
185. breast milk has 2 proteins: whey and casein
186. formula milk has way more casein than breast milk and makes it harder to digest
187. inflammatory breast cancer = redness, peau d'orange, cancer cells located in skin lymphatics
188. pregestational diabetes associated with miscarriage and congenital anomalies , GESTATIONAL IS NOT AT RISK
189. gestational diabetes increased risk for c section, preeclampsia, baby can get macrosomia, hypoglycemia, hyperbilirubinemia, childhood obesity

190. fasting target = <95 mg/dL
191. 1 hour postprandial = <140 mg/DL
192. 2 hour postprandial = <120 mg/DL
193. C section should be considered in diabetics with fetus weight of 4500 g+ due to shoulder dystocia risk
194. GDM first line = diet, second line = insulin
195. most common pregestational diabetes congenital abnormalities = cardiac and NTD
196. incongruent fundal height w/ age next step = US
197. RH negative mom next step = RhoGAM at 28 weeks
198. urine culture with GBS strep = treat with ampicillin, penicillin IV prophylaxis in labor
199. prego Pap smear ASCUS next step = repeat pap smear postpartum
200. normal ABG = respiratory alkalosis with partial metabolic compensation
201. pregnant = plasma volume, CO, GFR increased
    1. Hb down, PLT down, WBC up
202. lower esophageal sphincter is weaker -> GERD
203. advanced maternal age = 35+ years old at delivery
204. normal findings in pregnancy = glycosuria secondary to high GFR
205. PCO2 at 40 is actually considered CO2 retention in pregnancy aka respiratory failure
206. US if fundal height doesn't match age by 3+ cm
207. TdAP vaccine = given every pregnancy, even if previously given
208. neonatal Hep b infection leads to cirrhosis and HCC
209. Tdap vaccine is killed vaccine safe in pregnancy give between 28 and 36 weeks to elicit IgG response to passive transmission to fetus

GYNECOLOGY

1. breast cancer screening = 40 yo+, annual mammography
2. dtap booster every 10 years
3. osteoporosis screening = 65 yo+
4. HPV vaccine can be taken age 9-26 any time in here
5. herpes zoster vaccine = 60 yo
6. pneumococcal vaccine = 65+ yo
7. meningococcal vaccine = 19-21 yo in college or in residence
8. pap smear starts at age 21 and every 3 years after that
9. HIV pt pap smear = every year
10. if hysterectomy, no need to do pap smear anymore
11. smoking inhibits ability to clear HPV
12. estrogen replacement therapy for short term effective for treating hot flashes
13. menopause = ovarian failure for 12 months, after age 40 yo
14. premature ovarian failure = menopause before age 40
15. AMH drop = antimullerian hormone is earliest marker to indicate decreased ovarian reserve
16. prolactinoma -> suppress gnrh -> suppress LH FSH -> low estrogen -> osteoporosis
17. hypothyroidism -> high TRH -> stimulation of prolactin -> hyperprolactinemia -> shut down gnrh/lh/fsh -> low estrogen -> osteoporosis
18. female athlete triad = eating disorder + amenorrhea + osteoporosis
19. most common location of osteoporosis fracture = thoracic spine compression fracture = think kyphosis
20. osteoporosis prevention = weight bearing exercise, calcium, vitamin D
21. anyone with secondary amenorrhea = rule out pregnancy b hcg

22. most common post rape bugs = trichomonas, chlamydia, gonorrhea, hep b, hiv, syphillis
    1. antidotes = metro, azithro, ceftriaxone, hep B IG + vaccine
    2. check pregnancy and HIV prophylaxis too
    3. check life threatening injuries first
    4. serology testing for HIV syphilis Hep B
23. most effective form of emergency contraception is copper IUD
24. oral emergency contraceptive pills = progestin only (if copper IUD contraindicated)
25. rape trauma syndrome 2 phases:
    1. acute phase = body aches, poor appetite and sleeping and emotional distress
    2. delayed phase = nightmares, flashbacks, somatic symptoms
26. before ordering emergency contraception, u need to do a pregnancy test
27. hysterectomy prone to ureter injury by staple or cauterizer
28. post hysterectomy ureter injury appears similar to pyelonephritis, if ureter gets cut, urine leaks into peritoneum and irritates GI and causes n/v
    1. after hysterectomy or oophorectomy, patient develops fever + flank pain = suspect ureter injury
29. cardinal ligament = anchors cervix to side wall = carries UTERINE ARTERIES
30. infundibular pelvic ligament aka suspensory ligament = carries OVARIAN VESSELS
31. percutaneous nephrostomy = placing stent in the renal pelvis to open it up = used when febrile kidney stones
32. 5 W's of post op fever: wi wa wo wa wo
    1. wind = pneumonia, atelectasis = ~day 1
    2. water = UTI = ~day 3

3. wound = ~day 5
4. walking = DVT or PE = ~day 7
5. wonder drugs = iatrogenic = ~day 9 (or 7+)
6. wabscess = ~days 10+

33. vaginal vault/cuff prolapse/stress incontinence rx
    1. first line = kegel
    2. second line = pessary
    3. third line = surgical anchoring to sacral ligaments like sacrospinous, uterosacral, sacrocolpopexy

34. pessary = a device that pushes all the walls outwards so that the bladder and roof can't collapse, they are like structural beams

35. 4 types of pelvic organ prolapse (POP) = think of all the walls of the vagina, if one side is too soft, results in a prolapse
    1. cystocele = bladder herniates against anterior wall too soft
    2. rectocele = rectum herniates against back wall to soft
    3. enterocele (central) = top too soft (can be uterus or post hysterectomy)
    4. paravaginal (lateral) = levator ani too slack

36. urethral hypermobility = when Q tip rotates on valsalva = stress incontinence

37. urethra not supported -> q tip rotates on valsalva = urethral hypermobility

38. urinary incontinence = anterior defect = cystocele

39. bulging mass = central defect = vaginal vault prolapse/uterine prolapse

40. constipation = posterior defect = rectocele; relieved with DRE

41. fibroids -> constipation by external compression of rectum

42. evisceration = exposed bowel to the outside because wound broke open
    1. tx for wound evisceration = cover bowel with sterile sponge soaked in saline and go to OR + abx

43. fascial disruption = crack in fascia that causes fluid to leak out into skin, continuous lots of flow draining, salmon pink color
    1. tx = abdominal binder + go to OR
44. subQ/hematoma/wound infection = usually red and tender and febrile
    1. tx = open wound + drain pus + abx
45. urine and peritoneal/lymph fluid can look the same, CREATININE TEST helps u tell if its urine or not
46. overflow incontinence causes = diabetes or spinal cord injury
    1. tx = intermittent catheterization
47. urge incontinence tx = bladder training/oxybutynin anticholinergic
48. stress incontinence occurs when the proximal urethral sphincter falls below the pelvic diaphragm
49. when u have a normal bladder positioning, a cough will compress both the bladder and internal urethra so that there is no spillage, but if the urethra is below the pelvic diaphragm, then the cough will only compress the bladder and cause u to leak urine
50. dx of vesicovaginal fistula = colored dye in the bladder, continuous wet vagina flow
51. normal post void volume <100 ml/cc
52. urinary incontinence should rule out UTI first
53. signs of PID = red cervix, tender cervix, uterus tenderness, adnexal tenderness, fever, dyspareunia cuz cervix is inflamed, pelvic mass on US (tubo ovarian abscess), discharge
54. gonorrhea chlamydia target the endocervix columnar cells -> friable cervix -> postcoital bleeding
55. PID often has mucopurulent yellow discharge from cervix MOST LIKELY CHLAMYDIA
    1. next step = SPECULUM TO CHECK IF CERVIX OR VAGINA

56. trichomonas = VAGINITIS, strawberry red cervix, green frothy discharge, also can cause mucopurulent discharge too, tx = metro
57. gonorrhea = intracellular diplococci gram-
    1. migratory arthritis
    2. oral sex can cause infect pharynx too -> pustules/pharyngitis
    3. painful pustules on skin
58. outpatient PID tx = ceftriaxone + doxy
59. inpatient PID tx = cefotetan + doxy
60. PID -> tubo ovarian abscess (anaerobes mostly)
    1. tx = clindamycin or metronidazole
    2. US shows ovarian or adnexal mass
    3. can rupture
    4. no need to drain abx is good enough
61. IUD increases risk of PID
62. gold standard most accurate method for dx PID = laparoscopic
63. YELLOW CERVIX DISCHARGE = CHLAMYDIA >>> gonorrhea
64. long term sequelae of PID = infertility, ectopic, chronic pelvic pain
65. PID + adnexal mass = tubo ovarian abscess
    1. dx = sonography
    2. tx = abx covering anaerobes
66. pelvic pain worsened with menses = endometriosis, adenomyosis, or chronic pelvic pain
67. chronic pelvic pain syndrome = idiopathic somatic sx disorder of pelvis
    1. tx = NSAID for 3 mo or OCP
    2. tx refractory = laparoscopy
68. pain that varies throughout menstrual cycle = endometriosis or adenomyosis

69. painful uniformly enlarged boggy uterus = adenomyosis
70. refractory endometriosis tx = hysterectomy with BSO (bilateral salpingo oophorectomy)
71. primary dysmenorrhea = pain starts usually starts with first period, ELEVATED endometrial PROSTAGLANDIN F2 -> UTERINE CONTRACTIONS -> PAIN
    1. tx = NSAIDS
72. fishy odor + white discharge = bacterial vaginosis = gardnerella
    1. vaginosis = gram variable anaerobes
    2. tx = metronidazole or clindamycin
    3. KOH whiff +
    4. vaginal pH >4.5
    5. loss of lactobacilli allows for anaerobes to take over
73. metronidazole + alcohol = disulfiram like reaction
74. CANDIDA IS ACIDIC PH <4.5 ONLY ONE AND KOH-
75. vaginosis AND trichomonas both are KOH whiff+
76. trichomonas = anaerobic protozoa with flagella
77. DIABETES associated with persistent candida infection hard to control
78. itching + burning + after abx + thick cheesy discharge = CANDIDA
79. trichomonas tx = metronidazole oral 1 dose (NOT VAGINAL cuz it can hide in the urethra or skene glands)
80. bacterial vaginosis is associated with preterm delivery, postpartum endometritis, PID
81. syphilis serology = RPR or VDRL, if those are negative then u do a DARKFIELD MICROSCOPY just in case the antibodies aren't there yet
    1. syphilis dx = FTA ABS (will remain positive for life)
    2. tx = IM PENICILLIN LONG ACTING
82. if older patient, and chronic vaginal ulcer, should consider squamous cell carcinoma

83. chancre has clean indurated hard edges
84. chancroid has ragged edges, necrotic base
    1. h ducreyi g- rod
    2. school of fish appearance
    3. tx = azithromycin or ceftriaxone
    4. dx = culture or biopsy
85. neurosyphilis dx = lumbar puncture tx = IV penicillin
86. lymphogranuloma venereum = chlamydia trachomatis l1l2l3 = painless small ulcers + buboes that are painful
    1. dx = culture
    2. tx = doxycycline
87. granuloma inguinale = klebsiella = inguinal granulomas
    1. large painless many ulcers with no lymphadenopathy + ulcerated buboes
    2. has donovan bodies = intracellular inclusions inside of macrophages
    3. tx = doxycycline or tmp smx
88. if syphilis titers go down and then go back up it is because of REINFECTION
89. if RPR titers do not fall after treating next step = LP = it is possibly NEUROSYPHILIS
90. number 1 cause of UTI = e coli
91. tx for e coli cystitis = 1)tmp smx 2) nitro 3) fq; pregnant = 1) amoxicillin 2) cephalosporin 3) nitro
92. URETHRITIS = sterile pyuria = wbc+ bugs-
    1. next step = urethral swab -> gram stain + culture + NAAT
    2. think G/C
93. interstitial cystitis = sterile pyuria + relieved with urination
94. urethral syndrome = idiopathic urethritis = negative urine culture + negative urethral culture + dysuria
95. UTI triad aka cystitis triad = dysuria, urgency, frequency

96. gross hematuria = suspicious for nephrolithiasis

97. older painless gross hematuria = RCC or bladder cancer

98. asymptomatic bacteriuria in pregnant woman SHOULD ALWAYS BE TREATED PROPHYLACTICALLY

99. pyelonephritis pregnant = ceftriaxone

100. once a pregnant woman stabilizes her pyelonephritis, she should stay on prophylactic NITROFURANTOIN for the rest of the pregnancy

101. teratogenic antibiotics = Countless SAFe Moms Take Really Good Care

    1. clarithromycin

    2. sulfas

    3. aminoglycosides (kidney)

    4. fluoroquinolones (bones/tendons)

    5. metronidazole, macrolides

    6. tetracycline (teeth)

    7. ribavirin

    8. griseofulvin

    9. chloramphenicol (bm suppression)

102. Leiomyoma tx = 1) NSAID OR PROGESTIN 2) myomectomy/hysterectomy 3) embolization

103. tx of symptomatic anemia fibroids = hysterectomy

104. description of leiomyoma = non tender, midline irregular mass that moves together with the cervix when the cervix is moved

105. dx of fibroid = US

106. leiomyoma hysterectomy = when sx persist even after pharm and patient no longer wants kids, otherwise do myomectomy

    1. myomectomy = when sx leiomyoma and desires future pregnancy

107. if patient refuses surgical resection of fibroids, do

UTERINE ARTERY EMBOLIZATION

108. very fast growth of fibroid is suspicious for LEIOMYOSARCOMA

109. rapid growth of tumor + prior radiation exposure to pelvis = leiomyosarcoma

110. threatened abortion = spotting during <20 weeks pregnancy, baby can still survive tho, follow up bhcg in 48 hours

111. complete abortion = follow up bhcg until 0 to make sure that everything has expelled, passage of tissue + end of cramping (no more uterus contractions) + closed cervix = complete abortion

112. missed abortion = no bleeding no cramping but baby is dead

113. most common cause of spontaneous abortion = chromosomal/karyotope abnormality

114. hcG = glycoprotein = secreted by syncytiotrophoblast

115. hcg above 1500 and cant see baby on TVUS = ectopic most likely

116. progesterone level >25 = normal intrauterine pregnancy

117. for viable pregnancy check progesterone level <5 = baby dead

118. non viable pregnancy dx = slow hcg rise OR progesterone <5

119. stable vitals + ectopic pregnancy mgmt = MTX

120. unstable vitals + ectopic mgmt = surgical

121. tx of incomplete abortion = d&c to prevent infection

122. laparoscopy = confirms ectopic

123. molar pregnancy = vaginal spotting, super elevated b hcg, US snowstorm, super big uterus, trophoblastic tissue only

124. TVUS can detect pregnancy at 5 weeks

125. sx ruptured ectopic pregnancy aka syncope = laparoscopic

surgery right away b/c emergency

126. OCP best for anemia, dysmenorrhea, ovarian cysts, endometriosis
     1. risk of OCP = hepatic adenoma, breast cancer, MI, DVT, PE, Stroke, HTN
127. copper IUD = damages ovum
     1. disadvantages = heavy bleeding
     2. CI = wilson disease
128. Myth busted: OCP DOES NOT cause depression or weight gain
129. Depot injectable SE = DEPRESSION + WEIGHT GAIN + OSTEOPOROSIS
130. copper IUD works up to 5 days within intercourse
131. think of OCP as decreasing cycles of menses which preserves the endometrium and ovaries from getting beat up eg less cancer
132. incomplete abortion -> retained products -> sepsis
133. septic abortion next step = stabilize -> broad abx -> IVF -> D&C again
     1. septic abortion story line: incomplete abortion -> d&c not thorough -> parts remain -> vagina bacteria colonize retained products -> contractions, bleeding, fever -> tx is abx, fluids, d&c again
     2. septic abortion has foul smelling discharge
     3. infection is polymicrobial/anaerobic
     4. septic abortion abx tx = clindamycin + gentamicin
     5. refractory septic abortion that doesnt work with abx and d&C = hysterectomy
     6. septic abortion can lead to necrotizing metritis with gas pockets in the myometrium -> hysterectomy
134. abx for 4 hours before u do a d&c to allow abx to get peak efficacy

135. listeria infection = dark green amniotic fluid, gram+ rods
   1. chorioamnionitis via blood thru placenta
   2. dx = amniocentesis
   3. tx = IV ampicillin
   4. listeria is the only kind of chorioamnionitis where u dont need to deliver right away because membrane intact, other chorioamnionitis u should deliver right away
136. firm, round rubbery, mobile, non tender mass = fibroadenoma
137. ANY mass on the breast will need to be biopsied
   1. young pt = US (sees thru dense tissue better) <30 yo
   2. older pt = mammography (less density in older ppl) >30 yo
138. 3 types of biopsy
   1. FNA = for low risk pt = syringe that pulls out loose individual cells
   2. core biopsy = sample preserves cellular architecture see histo
   3. excisional = removes entire mass
139. LCIS biopsy = excisional biopsy
140. risky signs for malignancy = fixed mass, nipple retraction (invasion of cooper's suspensory ligaments), bloody nipple discharge
141. most common malignant tumor = invasive ductal carcinoma
142. fibrocystic changes = multiple lumps n bumps, cord like
   1. exaggerated response to estrogen
   2. breast painful engorgement prior to menses
   3. tx = stop coffee, take NSAID, take OCP
   4. still need to biopsy to make sure
   5. usually premenopausal

143. BRCA 1 = ONE = chromosome 17
144. BRCA 2 = TWO = chromosome 13
145. intraductal papilloma = unilateral bloody discharge
146. galactocele = obstruction leads to pockets of milk; tx = nsaids, breast pumping if still feeding
147. inflammatory breast cancer red skin because cancer cells obstruct lymph drainage and it causes swelling
148. paget disease of breast = rash over nipple most likely underlying adenocarcinoma
149. premenopausal breast cancer or bilateral breast cancer is suspicious for BRCA
150. BRCA breast cancer screening = MRI at age 25
151. with a breast mass, even if there is normal imaging, u still gotta do a biopsy
152. age is most important risk factor for cancer
153. ACOG guidelines = age 40 = yearly breast exam + mammography
154. ashkenazi jews are high risk BRCA carriers
155. when breast cyst fluid is yellow and mass disappears, then fluid can be discarded and no further therapy needed, f/u in 4 weeks
156. if fluid from breast is bloody, u should send it in for analysis
157. a mass that persists after aspiration should be biopsied
158. suspicious mammogram findings = small cluster of calcifications, ill defined border mass
159. triple negative = estrogen, progesterone, her 2 negative = poor prognosis
160. her2/neu is most aggressive breast cancer
161. d&c -> amenorrhea = asherman
    1. dx gold standard = hysteroscopy (or hysterosalpingogram or saline infused US can work too)
    2. negative progesterone challenge test = no withdrawal

bleeding = no endometrial sloughing off

   3. hysterosalpingogram of asherman = irregular filling of fluid

   4. tx = hysteroscopy and remove of the adhesions

162. most common cause of 2ndary amenorrhea = pregnancy

   1. other common causes = hypothyroid, prolactinemia, sheehan, premature ovarian failure

163. galactorrhea = hyperprolactinemia

164. hot flashes = ovarian failure

165. assessment for 2ndary amenorrhea algorithm: 1) b hcg + tsh + prl

   1. do pregnancy test

   2. check TSH and prolactin

   3. progestin challenge test

      1. if bleeding = PCOS/anovulation

      2. if no bleeding check pituitary ovarian axis FSH LH Estrogen

         1. if all 3 low = hypogonadotropic hypogonadism

         2. if estrogen low FSH LH high = ovarian failure

         3. if all 3 normal = asherman

166. breast feeding -> incr prolactin -> feedback shut down of LH/FSH -> shut down of axis -> no ovulation -> low estrogen

167. galactorrhea next step = check BHCG, TSH check PRL

   1. TRH acts as prolactin releasing hormone PRH

   2. causes for galactorrhea = pregnancy, prolactinoma, breast stimulation, antipsychotics, hypothyroidism

   3. galactorrhea on microscopy = fat droplets

   4. MRI for prolactinoma dx

   5. prolactinoma tx first line = cabergoline/bromocriptine

6. pregnancy -> elevated prl -> galactorrhea
7. bromocriptine safe in pregnant woman with prolactinoma
8. galactorrhea + no other explanation + normal menses = observation
9. oligomenorrhea + galactorrhea = pregnancy test

168. obese + irregular cycles = PCOS
169. PCOS associated with diabetes
170. tx for sheehan = replace hormones synthetically
171. PCOS complications = endometrial cancer + metabolic syndrome + cvd
    1. things to evaluate = 1) pelvic US follicles 2) TEST/DHEAS levels
172. virilism = acne + temporal balding + clitoromegaly + deep voice (DOES NOT HAPPEN IN PCOS, HAPPENS IN SERTOLI LEYDIG)
173. hirsutism = hairyness
174. 17 hydroxyprogesterone levels (elevated) measured to rule out CAH
175. PCOS benefits of OCP = regulate periods, stop endometrial hyperplasia, increase SHBG which will bind to excess androgens, and suppress ovary hormone production
    1. BMI <30 and wants to get pregnant tx = clomiphene
    2. BMI >30 and wants to get pregnant tx = anastrozole -> less estrogen -> increase LH/FSH -> ovulate
176. giant 10 cm ovarian mass = sertoli leydig tumor
177. giant 30 cm ovarian mass = mucinous ovarian tumor pseudomyxoma peritonei = ascites
178. Sertoli Leydig Ovarian Tumor
    1. makes androgen
    2. 10 cm ovary + clitoromegaly + recent rapid hair growth = SERTOLI LEYDIG TUMOR

    3. next step = CT surgical cancer staging

179. PCOS vs Sertoli Leydig

    1. PCOS is slow onset since first period ever …hirsutism

    2. Sertoli Leydig is very sudden …virilization

180. VIRILIZATION/CLITORMEGALY/VOICE DEEPENING DOES NOT HAPPEN IN PCOS

181. young girl who is going thru puberty way too early + huge 10 cm ovarian mass = granulosa theca tumor

    1. sertoli leydig = male features

    2. granulosa theca = female features

182. family hirsutism dx = ONLY HAIR is the problem nothing else, labs normal

183. sertoli leydig rx = surgical removal

184. most common cause of ambiguous genitalia = 21 hydroxylase deficiency CAH

185. 17 hydroxylase def = low cortisol and low sex but high aldo

186. 11 hydroxylase def = high 11 DOC = aldosterone effect; low cortisol, high androgen

187. Turner Syndrome

    1. next step to dx = FSH levels high

188. no secondary sex characteristics after age 12 female, 14 male= delayed puberty

189. secondary sex characteristics before age 8 female, 9 male = precocious puberty

190. most common cause of precocious puberty = idiopathic

    1. rx = gnrh agonist = leuprolide to shut down the axis

191. turner syndrome = remains prepubertal all the way til adult life, looks like a kid

    1. short height, webbed neck, shield chest, low ears

    2. streak ovary = fibrotic ovary-like tissue that doesn't work

    3. coarctation, bicuspid valve, horseshoe kidney

192. hypogonadotropic hypogonadism top causes = poor eating, excessive exercise, stress

193. tx for turner = hormonal supplements + growth hormone

194. presence of pubic hair = testosterone receptor is working good = good for AIS dx = if pubic hair, unlikely to be androgen insensitivity syndrome

195. mullerian agenesis = has good pubic hair growth (AIS does not)

196. primary amenorrhea + no secondary sex characteristics = turner
    1. turner shield chest, no breasts

197. AIS the testicles are taken out after puberty when it has increased chance of cancer

198. NO UTERUS + GOOD HAIR GROWTH = MULLERIAN = normal labs
    1. karyotype 46xx testosterone normal

199. NO UTERUS + NO HAIR GROWTH = AIS
    1. karyotype 46xy testosterone elevated

200. tx of septate uterus = hysteroscopic resection, dx = hysterosalpingogram; at risk for recurrent loss of pregnancy

201. AIS breast growth mechanism = excess unused testosterone gets converted to estrogen by aromatase and hits the breasts
    1. that's why dudes on roids get breasts

202. in turner 46xy or AIS 46xy, the gonad becomes malignant because of the Y chromosome
    1. turner 45XO streak ovary does not become malignant tho

203. kallman = loss of gnrh neurons, no smell, small testicles, delayed puberty

204. 3 D's of endometriosis = dysmenorrhea, dyspareunia, dyschezia

205. infertility = cannot get pregnant after 1 yr of trying, first

thing to assess = semen analysis

206. endometriosis -> interferes with ovulation -> incr risk for infertility

207. obesity -> excess estrogen -> endometrial hyperplasia -> cancer

208. most common cause of postmenopausal bleeding = atrophy

209. U MUST RULE OUT ENDOMETRIAL CANCER IN ANY POST MENOPAUSAL WOMAN WITH BLEEDING

210. description of endometrial cancer = endometrial hyperplasia with cellular atypia = CANCER

211. tx for endometrial cancer
    1. hysterectomy + BSO
    2. omentectomy in stage 2 because it can metastasize
    3. lymph node sampling
    4. peritoneal washing

212. pelvic irradiation associated with leiomyosarcoma

213. postcoital bleeding + foul discharge + smoking hx + hx of STD = cervical cancer

214. postcoital spotting = suspicious for cervical cancer

215. HPV and HIV are also risk factors for cervical cancer

216. HPV vaccine = killed = give age 9-26
    1. strains 6 and 11 = warts
    2. strains 16 and 18 = cervical cancer

217. cervical cancer metastasis can block the ureters and cause hydronephrosis main cause of death in cervical cancer

218. genital wart = condyloma acuminata

219. paps 21 yo every 3 years, stop paps at age 65

220. atypical glandular cell on pap next step = colposcopy + endocervical curettage + endometrial biopsy

221. at age 30 pap smear can do 2 ways:
    1. standard every 3
    2. pap + hpv every 5

222. majority of cervical cancers are squamous type
223. ovarian cancer
    1. ascites + cancer sx = ovarian cancer
    2. ascites compresses the bowels so u will get full quickly, bloating and have problems with bowel movements
    3. staging of ovarian cancer and endometrial cancer is same: hysterectomy with bso, omentectomy, lymph node biopsy, peritoneal washing
224. <30 yo most common tumor is teratoma -> ovarian torsion
225. vulvar cancer = itchy + ulcer/mass
226. 3 types of ovarian cancers
    1. epithelial = serous, mucinous
    2. germ cell = stem cell type = teratoma, embryonal carcinoma, dysgerminoma
    3. sex cord/stromal = hormonal = granulosa, sertoli leydig (SOLID TUMORS on US)
227. dx of teratoma = US, hyperechoic pockets, torsion is common, calcifications
    1. tx = oophorectomy or cystectomy
228. septations, solid components are usually neoplastic
229. mass >2cm in a prepubertal girl should be removed, need to take it more seriously cuz its unusual
230. labia minora white and thin + fibrosis/retraction of clitoris + vulvar itching = lichen sclerosus
    1. next step = punch biopsy
    2. therapy = corticosteroid topical
    3. lichen sclerosus histo = elongation of rete pegs, hyperkeratosis, thin epidermis
    4. itching is worse at night is a good clue
    5. cigarette paper look
    6. scarring can cause retraction of clitoris or fusion of the opening of the vagina can also fuse anus

7. hygiene is key to relieving sx = non irritating soaps, cotton underwear
8. lichen sclerosis left untreated can become sq cell cancer
231. bartholin gland abscess tx = incision and drain + marsupialize or balloon catheter to maximize drainage = polymicrobial bugs
    1. women over 40 yo+ should get biopsy cuz it could be cancerous
232. tx of vulvar cancer = removal of lesion and also inguinal lymph nodes = usually squamous cell
233. postmenopausal woman with painful sex = atrophy
    1. tx = topical estrogen

QUESTION BANKS

1. acute fatty liver disease of pregnancy = happens in last trimester, n/v + hypoglycemia + liver enzymes
2. hyperemesis gravidarum = hypochloremic hypokalemic hypoglycemic metabolic alkalosis
3. paget of breast and vulva = adenocarcinoma
4. pregnant woman glucose goals:
    1. fasting <95
    2. 1 hour <140
    3. 2 hour <120
5. secondary amenorrhea workup:
    1. first bhcg
    2. then prolactin and TSH
6. always rule out pregnancy with b hcg before u do any imaging
7. hydatidiform mole signs:
    1. preeclampsia <20 weeks
    2. profuse vomiting hyperemesis
    3. overly enlarged uterus
8. fitz hugh curtis = PID + RUQ pain + fever + hypotension
9. endometritis = uterine tenderness + foul lochia + fever
10. septic abortion = unsterile abortion = give D&C + ABX
11. screening for gonorrhea/chlamydia = <25 yo and high risk for infection such as new partner or previous STI
12. ovarian cancer = septated mass with solid components on US
13. BPP of 0-4 = immediate delivery
14. unclear 4-8 BPP = repeat BPP in 24 hours
15. BPP of 8-10 = good = no hypoxia = repeat in 1 week ?
16. doppler with no FHR = maybe baby died = do transabdominal US to confirm
17. NST = doppler FHR vs. Time (good = 15/15 2 in 20 = 15 HR increase for 15 seconds x2 episodes in 20 minute observation

period)

18. chorioamnionitis = fever + fetal tachycardia + uterine tenderness + purulent foul smelling discharge + prolonged ROM

    1. abx + deliver baby vaginally immediately

19. syphilis tx = IM Penicillin G

20. lichen sclerosus dx = punch biopsy; can become SCC

    1. rx = steroid

21. greatest risk factors for breast cancer = age >50 + family hx

22. tx for primary dysmenorrhea = NSAID or OCP

23. Q Tip test = to dx urethral hypermobility/stress incontinence = >30 degree angle with bearing down

24. first line tx stress incontinence = kegels

25. inevitable abortion and unstable = D&C cuz drugs take too long

26. inevitable abortion and stable = medical misoprostol

27. ruptured ovarian cyst = acute abdomen pain, dx US free fluid in peritoneum

    1. if stable = outpatient analgesics

    2. if unstable = surgical

28. Anovulation = ovaries make hormone but cant rupture, normal lh fsh

29. Pof = ovary doesn't make hormone or ovulate anymore high lh fsh

30. intrahepatic cholestasis = third trimester, super itchy palms and soles at night, increase bile acids, liver enzymes in the thousands, rx = ursodiol, deliver 1 week early

31. acute fatty liver of pregnancy = third trimester, n/v, hypoglycemia, liver failure; deliver immediately

32. PUPPP = pruritic urticarial papules and plaques of pregnancy = rash in the abdominal striae, benign rx = steroids

33. magnesium toxicity = hyporeflexia, respiratory depression

1. CI in renal failure b/c excreted by kidneys
2. tx = ca gluconate
34. PCOS = elevated testosterone, estrogen, first line tx = weight loss
35. endometriosis = chronic pelvic pain that worsens right before period, UTEROSACRAL LIGAMENT THICKENING/BUMPS
    1. tx = NSAID/OCP -> Laparoscopic Search
    2. ASSOCIATED WITH INFERTILITY
36. symmetric IUGR = genetics or torch infection
37. asymmetric IUGR = lack of nutrients or blood/hypoxia
38. healthy pregnant woman = incr plasma vol -> incr CO -> incr RBF -> incr GFR = PEE MORE + glycosuria ; physiologic anemia
39. PCOS = anovulation + obesity, bilaterally enlarged ovaries
    1. triad = hirsutism, irregular periods, polycystic ovaries on US
40. OCP INCREASED RISKS OF = VTE, HTN, HEPATIC ADENOMA, STROKE
41. at weeks 28 check/give = diabetes, rhogam, cbc (anemia)
42. at week 35-37 check = GBS test
43. adequate contraction = 200 montevideo units in 10 mins, approx contractions every 2-3 mins
44. Rhogam shots = at 28 weeks and again right after delivery
45. TSS = hypotension + macular rash involving palms and soles, look for hx of tampon or nose packing
    1. s aureus exotoxin -> super activation of t cells -> releases lots of cytokines
    2. IV fluids + abx
46. postpartum fever is normal within 24 hours after birth
47. hematocolpos = imperforate hymen tx = incision and drainage
48. decr fetal movement = do NST

49. no response NST = do BPP
50. if u dont hear FHR on doppler sonography U MUST CONFIRM WITH TRANSABDOMINAL ULTRASOUND to dx baby death
51. endometrial thickness >4mm = TOO THICK, should biopsy
52. previous preterm labor + short cervix = progesterone injection + cerclage, check TVUS of cervix length every week until 24 weeks
53. previous preterm labor + normal cervix = progesterone injection
54. no preterm labor + short cervix = vaginal progesterone
55. IUGR = less than 10th percentile
56. maternal obesity -> fetal macrosomia -> shoulder dystocia
57. fetal anemia = SINUSOIDAL HR
58. mag sulfate good up to 32 weeks
59. tocolytics good up to 34 weeks, after that is dangerous (close ductus arteriosus)
60. steroids good up to 37 weeks
61. primary dysmenorrhea = cramps during menses + normal exam
    1. rx = NSAID or OCP
62. DS = flat nose, rotated ears, sandal gap toes, hypotonia, epicanthic folds, protruding tongue, palmar crease, double bubble duodenum
63. recurrent first trimester losses are suspicious for lupus antiphospholipid/uterine anomaly; false positive VDRL; elevated PTT that does not correct with mixing studies
64. pregnant woman with pulmonary HTN = HIGH RISK FOR DEATH = bad cardiac output and oxygenation during pregnancy
65. oligohydramnios -> pulmonary hypoplasia
66. beta thalassemia = elevated HBA2 and elevated HBF
67. tx for lupus flare = corticosteroids

68. paroxetine can cause pHTN in the fetus
69. DS screening
    1. first trimester = beta hcg + nuchal + pappa
    2. second trimester = quad screen
    3. if any of those are +ve, u will confirm with chorionic villus sampling weeks 10-12 or amniocentesis week 15
70. preterm premature rupture of membranes abx = ampicillin + erythromycin
71. phosphatidylglycerol positive in vaginal fluid = fetal lungs are now mature enough
72. combined hormone therapy for menopause GREATEST RISK = BREAST CANCER
73. tamoxifen breast cancer therapy GREATEST RISK = ENDOMETRIAL CANCER
74. folate = 0.4 mg/day but if previous NTD kid = 4 mg/day

MISCELLANEOUS

1. 24 wks to 36+7 wks = preterm
2. 37 wks to 41+7 = term
3. 37 = term, 42 = post term
4. prolonged rupture of membranes = 18 hours+ of rupture until delivery (you have only 18 hours to get the baby out before it gets infectious)
5. ascending infection ROM = group b strep
6. prolonged rupture of membranes tx = ampicillin for baby protection
7. 20-28 weeks investigate 3 diseases: gestational diabetes, rh status, maternal anemia
8. PPH
    1. absent uterus = uterine inversion = tx with manual, tocolytics before to make it pliable + oxytocin after to contract
    2. boggy uterus = uterine atony = do a uterine massage
    3. firm uterus irregular endometrial stripe = retained placenta = do d+c or hysterectomy, f/u b hcg to make sure it all came out
    4. normal uterus = look for vaginal laceration = fix with sutures (clue = s/p forceps)
    5. normal uterus without laceration = look for DIC
9. NST non reassuring = no accelerations seen; next step = vibroacoustic stimulation to possibly wake him up; if vibroacoustic stimulation non reassuring next step = BPP
10. BPP score 0-2 = emergency c-section, BPP 8+ = reassure
11. 15/15 2 in 20 = 15 second 15 incr hr twice in 20 mins = good accels = reassuring NST
12. asx bacteriuria/uti for pregnant mom tx = amoxicillin or nitrofurantoin

13. pyelo in pregnant tx = ceftriaxone
14. TOGV A/W PREGESTATIONAL DIABETES
15. pregnant woman has increased requirement for thyroid and insulin replacement
16. preeclampsia severe features = 160/110 or evidence of end organ damage; next step = magnesium + deliver vaginally, timeline doesn't matter save mom
17. 2 types of 3rd trimester painful bleeding:
    1. uterine rupture = loss of fetal station is key sign, usually 2/2 pmh of c-section
    2. abruption = severe htn, mva; PAINFUL
18. 2 types of painless 3rd trimester bleeding = placenta previa and vasa previa, both tx with c section
19. group b strep manifestations = neonatal pneumonia, meningitis, chorioamnionitis, endometritis
20. blueberry muffin baby = rubella = cataracts, cardiac, deaf
21. 3 things that incr risk of DVT in OB/GYN population = estrogen from contraception, smoking, 35 yo+
22. cervical ca = post coital bleed, endometrial ca = post meno bleeding
23. ovarian cancer signs = ascites, weight loss, small bowel obstruction, hydronephrosis
24. hydatidiform mole signs = hyperemesis gravidarum, preeclampsia, big uterus
25. ASCUS options = do HPV or repeat in 6 months
    1. ascus + hpv positive -> colpo
    2. ascus + hpv negative -> go back to normal screens
    3. ascus + repeat in 6 months is positive -> colpo
    4. ascus + repeat in 6 months is negative = go back to normal screens
26. abnormal pap next step = colposcopy
27. abnormal colposcopy next step = excision

28. after colposcopy:
    1. if squamous cells -> leep or cryo
    2. if columnar cells -> conization
29. adnexal mass first step = TVUS
30. complete mole person needs to be on OCP for 12 months while u track bhcg to make sure that if it comes back up u know its a choriocarcinoma and not pregnancy
31. incomplete mole = 1 egg + 2 sperm, chromosomes 69
32. complete mole = empty egg shell + 1 sperm that splits into 2, chromosomes 46
33. PPH first line tx = uterine massage
    1. 2nd line = oxytocin
    2. 3rd line = balloon tamponade
    3. last line = surgery uterine artery ligation or hysterectomy or embolization
34. ectopic tx:
    1. no rupture = salpingostomy
    2. rupture = salpingectomy
    3. mtx = if <3cm fetus or b hcg <5000
35. most common causes of vaginal bleeding:
    1. pediatric = foreign body; next step = speculum exam under anesthesia
    2. reproductive = pregnancy, anatomy, dysfxnl uterine bleeding (PAD); next step = preg test
    3. postmenopausal = vaginal atrophy, endometrial cancer, cervical cancer next step = think endometrial biopsy/colposcopy
36. PCOS
    1. anovulation, high testosterone, hirsutism, obesity, u/s shows lots of follicles
    2. tx = weight loss + metformin, spironolactone for hairiness, ocp for bleeding

37. AIS has testicles not ovaries, no uterus, NO HAIR, amenorrhea
38. 2ndary amenorrhea algorithm:
    1. first step = bhcg, tsh, prl
    2. second step = Progesterone challenge
    3. third step = FSH/LH
39. infertility first step = work up male first = semen analysis
40. dx of ectopic pregnancy = TVUS + BHCG
41. retained placenta = ultrasound will show irregular endometrium
42. lichen sclerosus vs atrophic vaginitis = vaginal mucosa is pale and dry in atrophic vaginitis
    1. lichen sclerosis has white crusting almost like eczema/psoriasis/fungal
    2. lichen = ITCHY, atrophic = DRY
43. first visit prenatal = chlamydia, hiv, hepatitis b, syphilis, rubella, chickenpox
    1. pap, urine culture, urine protein, rho
44. ovarian teratoma high risk for ovarian torsion
45. hyperemesis gravidarum dx = urine ketones+
46. oxytocin OD can cause seizures 2/2 hyponatremia
    1. 3 se of oxytocin = hyponatremia, hypotension, tachysystole
47. spiral artery vasoconstriction -> preeclampsia, preterm delivery, abruption, iugr
48. pathognomonic sign for uterine rupture = goes from positive to negative station aka 0 to -3
49. postmenopausal woman with US ovarian cyst/mass next step = ca125 = helps evaluate if it is most likely to be benign or malignant
50. signs of ovarian torsion = ACUTE SUDDEN onset adnexal pain, severe, n/v
51. greatest risk for asx bacteriuria/uti = preterm delivery
52. ovarian torsion a/w a OVARIAN MASS

53. breast engorgement = BILATERAL = production exceeds release from breast = painful, swollen, NON erythema breast
    1. if no longer feeding tx = nsaids
    2. if still feeding = breast pumping
54. first sign of magnesium toxicity = diminished DTR
55. PREVIOUS PRETERM LABOR + SHORT CERVIX = CERCLAGE + PROGESTERONE
56. PREVIOUS PRETERM LABOR + NORMAL CERVIX = INJECTED PROGESTERONE ONLY
57. NO PRETERM LABOR + SHORT CERVIX = VAGINAL PROGESTERONE ONLY
58. hyperemesis gravidarum = check urine ketones, tx = b6 vitamin
59. thickened nuchal translucency = Down Syndrome
60. abortion = terminated fetus before 20 weeks old
61. betamethasone = mature fetus lungs used <37 weeks
62. magnesium sulfate = most common tocolytic AND seizure prophylaxis in preeclampsia used <32 weeks for protection from cerebral palsy
63. tocolytics used up to 34 weeks
64. pregestational diabetes = 4x more likely for preeclampsia (narrowing of spiral arteries), cardiac defects, malformation
65. gestational diabetes incr risk for macrosomia
66. macrosomia = 4500 G baby, normal is 2500
67. IUGR = bottom 10% of weight of babies
68. braxton hicks contractions = contractions without dilations
69. latent phase of stage 1 of labor = up to 6cm dilation
70. active phase of stage 1 of labor = 6cm to max dilation period
71. postcoital bleeding is cervical cancer until proven otherwise
72. bacterial vaginosis = gardnerella = gray discharge, fishy odor and no itching
73. trichomonas = green frothy and itchy with strawberry cervix

74. rx for both vaginosis and trichomonas = metronidazole

MEDICATIONS USED IN OB/GYN

1. pregnant pyelonephritis = CEFTRIAXONE
2. pregnant endometritis = clindamycin + gentamicin
3. pregnancy UTI = Amoxicillin, nitrofurantoin
4. tubo ovarian abscess = clindamycin + metronidazole
5. septic abortion = clindamicin + gentamicin
6. preterm premature rupture of membranes (PPROM) = ampicillin + erythromycin
7. toxoplasma mom = spiramycin
8. toxoplasma fetus = pyrimethamine + sulfadiazine
9. tocolysis = terbutaline, indomethacin, nifedipine, ritodrine, magnesium
10. homozygous factor V leiden mutation = LMW heparin
11. pulmonary edema = furosemide
12. uterotonic agents = oxytocin, misoprostol, ergotamine
13. tachysystole rx = terbutaline = beta 2 agonist
14. endometritis = ampicillin + gentamicin
15. mastitis abscess = dicloxacillin + drainage
16. GDM second line after refractory diet = insulin
17. inpatient PID = cefotetan + doxy
18. primary dysmenorrhea = NSAID
19. syphilis = IM penicillin
20. chancroid = azithro or ceftriaxone
21. neurosyphilis = IV penicillin
22. lymphogranuloma venereum chlamydia L1 L2 L3 = doxycycline
23. fibroid = NSAID or progestin
24. stable patient ectopic pregnancy (if <3cm fetus or b hcg <5000) = mtx
25. listeria = ampicillin IV
26. fibrocystic changes = decrease caffeine, NSAID, OCP, severe = danazol

27. prolactinoma = cabergoline/bromocriptine
28. PCOS tx = OCP
29. PCOS BMI<30 trying for a kid = clomiphene
30. PCOS BMI >30 trying for a kid = aromatase inhibitor
31. idiopathic precocious puberty = gnrh agonist = leuprolide
32. turner = estrogen for 3 years then OCP, and also GH (prevents tubular breasts)
33. male factor/tubal factor trying to get pregnant = in vitro fertilization
34. lichen sclerosus = topical steroids
35. vaginal atrophy painful sex = topical estrogen
36. lupus flare = corticosteroids
37. magnesium overdose antidote = calcium gluconate

About the Author:

Steven Vuu aka Dr. High Yield, is a general surgery resident at the University of Central Florida. He was born and raised in Vancouver, BC, Canada. He completed his medical degree at Ross University School of Medicine, finishing in the top 5% of his class, graduating with Summa Cum Laude (Highest Honors). He was a Dean's Honor Roll and Dean's List student in all 4 years of medical school and scored above 250 and 265 on the USMLE Step 1 and 2 CK exams, respectively. His Step 2 CK score was approximately in the 95th percentile worldwide. He was head

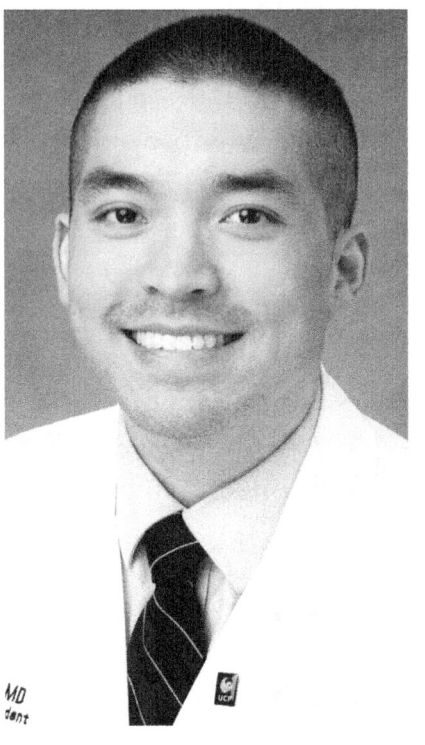

TA in medical school, and tutored full classrooms each week in preparation for their exams. There, he learned that he had helped many of his classmates increase their scores. This would eventually set the stage for his future in medical education. Before that, he graduated from The University of British Columbia in Vancouver, BC, Canada with a Bachelor's Degree in Science. During his spare time, he likes to make electronic music, work out, and watch movies.

Made in the USA
Monee, IL
13 August 2022

11556009R00036